Detox Cleanse

EXPRESS

Detox Cleanse

EXPRESS

Know How to Detox and Cleanse Your
Body Naturally

Theresa Holland & KnowIt Express

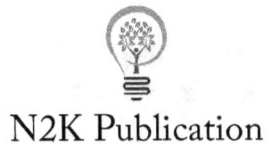

N2K Publication

ISBN 978-1-533-04145-6

Printed in the United States of America

First Edition

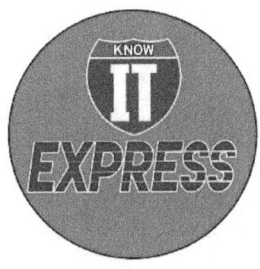

Welcome to the *Know It Express* - the express lane to knowledge!

To stay up-to-date, please be sure to sign up for **our newsletter** at http://www.KnowItExpress.com and follow us on social media:

https://www.facebook.com/KnowItExpress
https://twitter.com/KnowItExpress
https://plus.google.com/+KnowItExpress

Detox Cleanse Express

EXPRESS LANE

Detox Cleanse Express

Detox Cleanse Express

CHAPTER 1

Cleaning Out Your System

The Maintenance Of A Healthy Body

Your body is a **machine**. And just like a car, it requires *routine maintenance* to maintain optimal performance. After working for a long time, a car needs its oil changed and dirt drawn out from the pipes.

The same applies to the body. As you "drive" your body by eating and simply living, waste is generated. The main job of the **liver** and **kidneys** is to filter that waste, but depending on your lifestyle, lingering waste can remain over time and begin to accumulate.

Enter, the <u>detox</u>. A **detox** is a way of *cleansing the body of unwanted materials.*

Detox and cleansing are practices that have spanned throughout many centuries, and a good detox regimen can help you feel better and jump-start a healthier lifestyle.

- Now you might be wondering what is the difference between a detox and a cleanse. To put it simply, think of a cleanse as macro-cleaning done in a shorter time period (such as over the weekend) where you can immediately notice how much better your body feels afterward, while a detox takes more time in micro-cleaning toxins out of your system incrementally that have been built up over time, hence the prefix "de-" and "tox" together for "removal of toxins."

Feeling sluggish at work? Want to find out the food that's been giving you so many digestive troubles? Then a detox might be the <u>perfect option</u> for you.

Dextox In The Beginning

One of the *oldest forms* of detox is the **Ayurvedic method**, originating from India 5,000 years ago and considered to be one of the oldest medical practices.

In this technique, the body is fed with a **mono diet** that usually consists of *oatmeal* and *kitchari*. This diet is designed to give a temporary break to the digestive system, and when used in conjunction with a healing herb, it can give a boost to the body's immune system.

While detoxes have been performed for years, the importance and popularity has grown due to many factors. Many different forms of diets—many of which are detoxes—are being promoted in the media (as well as the doctor's office), and air pollution—something outside our control but always in the air we breathe—is a hot-button issue.

All of these factors combine to cause people to be hungry for their own personal "fix" to live their healthiest life, and a detox might be the answer.

CHAPTER 2

Determine When to Detoxify

Signs For Detoxification

Your car lets you know when it's time for an oil change. And, if you never change the oil, it will start to show signs of wear and tear. Your body will do the same. And if ignored, you can become used to those signs and continue trudging through life.

Thus, the importance of **detoxification** can't be emphasized enough. As *toxins* continue to build in your body, some of the following signs may begin to manifest:

- **Fatigue**: It's normal for everyone to become tired after strenuous work—mental or physical. But fatigue can follow you out of your sleep like a dark shadow for the better part of the day, making you feel and act somewhat sluggish. Once it gets to this point, more sleep may not solve the problem and you might need to search for the underlying cause.

- **Skin irritations**: If you suffer from skin irritation, you may know a few of the potential triggers. But there may be times when rashes and discoloration appear for no apparent reason. These ailments often occur in response to what's happening inside your body and not always due to what's going on around you.

- **Bloating:** We've all had those mornings where no amount of makeup or coffee will hide the bags under our eyes. Or a night of heavy eating or hard partying that has left behind nothing but a bloated feeling. When you see these signs more regularly, it's a good time to not ignore them and to go for a proper medical check.

- **Menstrual complications**: One indicator of a health disturbance in women is menstrual changes. This can take the form of delayed, irregular, or painful periods, discolored discharge, and so on.

- **Mental confusion**: When your body isn't running efficiently, your brain won't either. You may experience "brain fog," a lack of mental coordination, inability to focus, and so on.

Quiz: Time For A Detox

Below is a questionnaire developed to help you assess your need for a detox. To achieve the desired result, it is important you answer the questions as honestly as possible.

Your **rating** should be in the range of 1-4:
- 1 (never)

- 2 (maybe)
- 3 (sometimes)
- 4 (always)

1) Do you experience itching triggered by no known or observed cause?

2) Does your face remain puffy after an hour of waking?

3) Do you feel dizzy even when you're not hungry or feeling sleepy?

4) Do you experience blurry vision?

5) Do you notice rashes or discoloration of your skin?

6) Does your period of fatigue last longer than it used to?

7) Is there an increase in the re-occurrence of your low-grade infections?

8) Is there a sudden change in your libido or menstruation?

9) Is there a drop in your ability to focus on a particular task?

10) Do you experience loss of appetite?

After you have taken the test, add up your scores. If you scored 25 or above, it may be time for you to think about a detox.

CHAPTER 3

Ways to Detox Cleanse to Feel Better Now

Different Types Of Detoxifications

There are numerous <u>detox plans</u> available, and each has a specific target.

Some are **broad-based,** while others target **specific organs** of the body. It is therefore important to carry out a more streamlined test, unlike the one you did earlier. The streamlined test will focus on one particular area of the body and shut out the rest.

- For example, if you are aiming to detox the skin, you may *not* need to focus on issues related to concentration and mental ability.

The **condition-specific detoxes** aim to eliminate the cause of the symptoms you're facing. If you have more than one symptom, these can be done in order of importance to you.

It is always good to plan your procedure well and follow it to the letter for optimum result.

<u>Note</u>: Always check with your doctor before beginning any detox plan, as every person's body functions differently. We are not responsible for how your body may react.

Condition-Specific Detox 1: Fatigue

Too tired? When you have that sluggish feeling that you can't shake, then it may be time to try the steps below.

- You can start your detox right in the bathroom. Start by alternating your bath water with cold and hot water. The sharp changes in temperature can help circulation and can also cleanse the **lymphatic system.**

- The next step will be to work on your **diet.** All the good stuff must go--junk food, heavy carbohydrates, alcohol, and caffeine can all have a big impact on your energy level, and you won't feel a difference unless you make a commitment to cut them out completely. *Moderation is not the key here.*

- **Fiber, fiber, fiber.** Fiber helps empty the bowels and eliminate waste. Certain vegetables can be a good source of fiber and iron, which is helpful for blood formation. Healthier blood cells can help improve circulation, which can help remove toxins.

- **Water** is your friend. Simply taking a bath or taking a dip in a pool can help moisten the skin and refresh the pores.

- It might seem counterintuitive, but a little **exercise**—as little as 20 to 30 minutes a day will help to keep your blood flowing and help maintain nutrient flow to the skin.

Condition-Specific Detox 2: Distraction

Can't concentrate? You may get the impulse to grab a cup of coffee or an energy drink the moment you start losing focus, but brain fog might just be another way that your body is telling you to detox. Mental disorientation begins to occur when there are toxins and wastes in your system. The best thing to do at such points is to:

- Go for **multivitamins**, especially those with at least 200mg of vitamin C. A well-known naturopathic physician, **Michael T. Murray, ND,** from Bastyr

University in Seattle, said that most of the vitamins have strong antioxidant properties, which can play major roles in detoxification. He further stressed that nutrients such as *thiamine* and *foliate* help to remove heavy metals from the system.

- **Water-soluble fiber** enhances production of *bile* and should become a part of your diet. Water-soluble fiber can be obtained from oat, legumes, pears, and apples, to name a few. Refined foods (particularly sugars and alcohol) can block the flow of bile, which results in a medical condition called **cholestasis**. When this happens, fats are not easily metabolized and fat-soluble toxins become hard to eliminate.

- Take a **mental break.** *Yoga* is one exercise that can give your brain a rest. Studies have shown that wastes collect better when the body is in its relaxed state. Try 20-30 minutes of yoga every morning upon waking and see what difference it makes to your concentration and focus.

Condition-Specific Detox 3: Itch And Discomfort

Feeling itchy? The urge to scratch can come at any time, on any part of the body. Itchy sensations can be an indication that the liver (the body's detoxification center) is overwhelmed with toxins. Itching can be mild or intense depending on body type and the level of toxins. This phenomenon is also referred to as "liver itch" by some people. It can be difficult to fight the urge to scratch, but it can leave you with bruised or inflamed skin. Try the below steps instead:

- Itches are often an indication that the toxins are leaving the skin. **Clay** can help ease the itchy sensation and can help remove toxins from the skin. Just mix clay with clean water until you get a brown cream. <u>Note</u>: use clean water and heat up the cream to sterilize it. Carefully coat the itchy area with the clay mixture and, once it dries, peel or wash off.

- **Menthol** is also a great itch-reliever. If you don't have any, another alternative is to pluck a few peppermint leaves, crush them, and apply them onto the itchy areas.

- **Water, water, water.** If you can, drink a liter of water every two hours. Water is helpful with itchy skin to help keep the skin moisturized. Dry skin only makes itching worse and makes your skin brittle.

- Take a **cold bath** to end your day's therapy. In general, taking a bath helps to get rid of germs and waste, but a cold bath can help rid the muscles and capillaries of some of the toxins they contain.

Condition-Specific Detox 4: Pain And Ache

Can't get rid of aches and pains? Aches and pains are a common complaint of those detoxing, and one of the reasons is because toxins are moving out faster than the body is used to handling. But don't worry! The best remedy at such point is to detox those away, and relax the muscles and joints by following the steps below.

- **Activated charcoal** is made from Indian hardwood and comes in a capsule form. When ingested, the activated charcoal binds toxins and other unwanted gas molecules. And because of its large surface area, it can bind to toxins more effectively and adhere to them until they're eliminated in your waste.

- A **chemical bath** can help draw out toxins from your skin. *Sea salt* and *baking soda* have these abilities. Simply add a few tablespoons of either of these into a tub of warm water. Stir and sit still in it for at least 30 minutes. As water molecules and the molecules of the substances you added bombard your skin, they create a charge that draws those toxins out.

- Who doesn't love a **massage**? A very effective way to get rid of aches and pains, a massage can help eliminate toxins that block the blood vessels. You can massage yourself by running your hands on the aching points. Using your fingers, raise some of the skin in the area as if you're pinching yourself, but don't hold it so tight so that it hurts. Then push it down until you feel your bones. It's a similar movement to kneading dough. For areas your hands cannot reach (like your back), you can visit a masseuse or ask a friend to help you out.

CHAPTER 4

Renew Your Whole Body with Detox Cleanses

Sources Of Toxic Removal

If you desire to get rid of toxins, the first step would be to cleanse the organs responsible for the removal of the waste.

If the **excretory organs**—the skin, liver, and kidney—are running at their optimal performance, then you can help ward off some of the associated symptoms that occur when they're not working their best.

Organ-Specific Detox 1: Skin

The **skin** is the largest organ of the human body. Waste such as *urea* and *sodium* leave the skin through the tiny holes known as **sweat pores.** If you have severe skin irritation, or your skin reacts to just anything, there are some quick home remedies that can help you out.

For a skin cleanse, you'll need a cleanser, toner, detox mask, and oil serum. The proceeding steps outline a three-day process to refresh your skin. Take a before photo and watch the transformation!

- **Day 1:** Upon waking, rub your skin with **olive oil.** This helps to regulate oily skin. Allow the oil to stay on your skin for one to two hours, then wash it off. Follow with **toner** and **moisturizer.** Important note: During this three-day cleanse, do not wear any makeup.

- **Day 2:** Time to try out the detox mask. Mash canned **chickpeas** with a splash of water and a pinch of **turmeric acid**. Use this mixture to coat your skin on the areas you aim to detox. Wear it overnight if you can, but if not, two to three hours, should do the trick.

- **Day 3:** Use an **oil serum** to wash your skin. After finishing, take a look at your before photo to see if you notice any changes.

Organ-Specific Detox 2: Liver

The **liver** is the body's defense mechanism. When toxins enter the body, they are taken to the liver where they're filtered into waste to prevent them from causing more harm to the body. This workaholic organ is further strained by some harmful habits such as smoking, excessive intake of alcohol, consumption of fried or fatty foods, unsafe sex (which can result in hepatitis) and so on.

One wonderful property of the liver is that when it gets the desired break, it can heal itself. The following are some helpful practices that can keep your liver operating at its optimal health.

- **Herbal bitters:** These may not be your favorite, but your liver needs them. Bitter substances stimulate the production of bile. You can make bitters more palatable by adding them to **warm lemon juice** in the morning. The sourness of lemon juice can help activate nerves and hormones that can help with a better bowel movement. For an effective liver cleanse, make this a part of your breakfast for the next seven days.

- **Green veggies: Brassica** family sprouts—including cabbage, Brussels sprouts, and broccoli—contain **glucosinolates**. Glucosinolates are sulfur-containing compounds that can help protects the liver from damage and enhance its ability to eliminate excess hormones and toxins.

- **Turmeric: Turmeric** is so much more than the spice that makes your curries yellow. When ingested, turmeric has an anti-inflammatory effect and is good for fighting liver infections. Make this (a few sprinkles) part of your daily diet.

- **St. Mary's Thistle:** Also known as **milk thistle**, this supplement has antioxidant and antioxidant properties and is often used to treat liver problems.

- **Cut out the carbs and fatty foods:** Instead of pancakes, sandwiches, and pizza for breakfast, lunch, and dinner, try a **fruit fast** for a day or two. When you're done with that, incorporate meals that are rich in **antioxidant vitamins**—like vitamins C and E, and minerals such as zinc and selenium, which help aid in the metabolism of alcohol.

- **Stay hydrated:** During your liver cleanse (and beyond), it's important to drink lots of **water**. Water does to the liver what oil does to an engine—it takes nutrients to it and takes waste away from it. Lack of sufficient water increases your risk of *gallstones*, which occurs when the concentration of bile becomes too high in the gall bladder.

Organ-Specific Detox 3: Kidneys

More than just those bean-shaped organs in your abdomen, the **kidneys** work with your liver to eliminate excess water, sodium, and other toxins from the body. Inability of the kidney to perform adequate filtration can result in skin blemishes like acne, eczema, etc.

The kidney filters a large volume of water and blood daily, so, naturally, a kidney cleanse should come in the form of fluid so that it will get to the target destination. Some of the preparations that are very active in detoxifying the kidney are listed below.

- **Melon-Lime Juice:** Watermelon is more than 90% water and an amazing source of potassium, which can help with kidney stones. Squeeze two cups of **watermelon** and mix the juice with one cup of **lime**. Drink in the morning and wait for an hour before eating.

- **Cucumber-Carrot Juice:** This **cucumber** and **carrot** juice is a powerful detoxifier that helps to remove excess uric acid (one of the key causes of kidney stones) while also filling the body with a burst of nutrients. To prepare, wash one large cucumber and two carrots. Cut into smaller pieces and blend with 50ml of water. Sieve and enjoy your juice. One glass before you go to bed is adequate.

- **Cranberry Juice:** Researchers have shown that **cranberries** have the ability to fight urinary tract infection by decreasing the ability of bacteria to adhere to the bladder and urethra. Cranberries have also shown promise in mopping up excess calcium oxalate, which is one of the major causes of kidney stones. To make your own cranberry juice, get fresh cranberries and use a juicer to milk them. If you find that too much of a hard work and decide to buy it at the grocery store, make sure you find a brand without any added sugar, preservatives, or flavors.

- **Beet Juice:** *Beet it!* **Beet juice** is another very fine kidney detoxifier because of its betaine content, which is a great **phytochemical**. It's a good antioxidant and increases the acidity of urine. Beet juice helps to remove *calcium phosphate* and *struvite* which will not only help kidneys function better but also reduce the chances of kidney stones.

Organ-Specific Detox 3: Lungs

Lungs are responsible for getting rid of gases. You know we inhale oxygen (in combination with other gases) and exhale carbon dioxide through same means. Not all of these gases leave when we exhale. Some get stuck in the alveoli and find their way to the bloodstream through gaseous exchange between the blood and lungs.

Some of the ways to detox the lungs are the following.

- **Antioxidants are King:** Eat foods rich in **antioxidants,** as they enhance lung activity and can help improve the quality of breathing. Some of the foods rich in antioxidants are sweet potatoes, green tea, broccoli, spinach, grapes, etc.

- **No Smoking!** The smoke inhaled from tobacco has a lot of harmful substances, including those that cause damaging inflammation to the bronchial walls. *Eliminating any tobacco product* is the best way to detox the lungs.

- **Ventilation:** Detoxing the lungs goes beyond yourself, to your environment. Stay in a *well-ventilated environment.* This will help your lungs access cleaner air. Also, planting of **flowers** and

green vegetation will help to filter the air, or, if you are surrounded by a concrete jungle, a **HEPA filter** will do the trick.

- **Work Out: Aerobic exercise** makes the lung expand and contract faster. This helps to strengthen your lungs and helps them take and expel more air.

Organ-Specific Detox 4: Lymphatic System

The **lymphatic system** is a network of fluid-filled nodes, and its main function is removal of toxins and protection of the body from pathogens. It carries waste from the tissue into the bloodstream where its then removed. Therefore, a healthy individual owes a lot of thanks to his or her lymph network.

The lymphatic system can be detoxified by the following means.

- **Trampoline:** Remember jumping on this as a kid? Reinvent it now to help improve blood flow around the body. Researchers have shown it is good at detoxifying the lymphatic system.

- **Hanging Bat:** Sounds weird, right? But **inverting** actually stimulates the circulatory and lymphatic systems. It helps decompress the joints and brings blood and oxygen to the tissues.

- **Stay Hydrated:** The lymphatic system is estimated to be composed of **95% water.** When water is in short supply, lymphatic fluid's smooth movement is impeded. Stay hydrated by taking in lots of water.

- **Massage:** A good **lymphatic massage** helps the lymphatic system drain its toxins and stimulate movement of lymphatic fluids.

Total Body Detox

You need it all! A **total detox** is a holistic program that should take you a number of weeks to complete (and not just a day activity).

Jon Barron, a dedicated nutraceutical researcher and the director of Baseline of Health, provides instruction on the correct order and method to go about a total detox. **Colon detox** is very necessary and should come first, because if the colon is blocked, toxins from the liver and organs cannot be effectively removed.

There are two separate ways to perform a colon detox—an **oral colon detox** or using an **enema**.

- **Oral colon detox**: An oral colon detox involves a fruit fast for at least seven days. This means only eating fruit—watermelon, pawpaw, orange, lemon, apple, pineapple, banana etc.—for at least a week. There's no limit to the amount of fruits you can combine. The high water content of the fruits and its phytochemicals wash down impurities in your gut, while the high fiber makes its path smooth. Take this as much as you like for at least seven days.

- **Rectal colon detox**: Enemas have been used for thousands of years dating as far back as ancient Egypt 1550 B.C. This practice involves sending fluids into the rectum to directly clean the intestine. Note: It is always advised to do this under the supervision of a physician. The process starts with 1 liter of warm water, which can be customized with herbs and probiotics, which is passed into the rectum using a low-pressure pump.

CHAPTER 5

Perform Your On-going Internal Renewal

Tracking Progress

After learning about a variety of detox options, you should have a good idea of which you'd like to try. But the first step is commitment, and to help you keep committed, you need a **detox calendar**.

Here is a sample calendar that you can tweak as much as you like. The goal is to customize so you can stay true to it.

Sample Calendar for Total Detox

Days 1-7	Begin with colon detox. If this is your first detox, spend the first three days taking colon activator. On the fourth, you can begin taking the colon detoxifier.
Days 8-14	While still taking your colon detoxifier, begin your skin detox and run it simultaneously until the end day 14. Since the skin detox only takes three days, you'll run through it twice during this period).
Days 15-21	Wrap up your colon detox, and shift your focus to liver detox. Run this program for seven days.
Days 22-28	Wrap up liver detox, and begin your kidney detox. Run this program for seven days.

When you've completed your detox program, do you feel any difference in you body's physiology? Go back to the questionnaire on the first section, and take it again. If your score is still up to 25, consider seeking medical advice from a trained medical professional.

Staying Motivated

A detox calendar can help keep your detox on track—serving as a reminder and a diary—and will help you reach your ultimate goal. It should be bold and located in a place where you're sure to see it every day. Color coding is also a great idea.

Life is demanding, and priorities shift from day to day, so keeping your detox calendar in a place that you'll see it and updating it daily will make it easy to continue to follow your regimen.

A stare at your detox calendar will help you not to forget about your detox program. It's similar to placing your prescriptions in a pill box. When everything is clearly organized and labeled, following instructions is easier than ever.

Just as following and maintaining compliance with your prescriptions is important to the long-term maintenance of your health, following your detox schedule is an important piece of seeing the results you're looking for.

Another benefit of the detox calendar is monitoring your progress. You can make note of side effects felt, when you started to notice a difference, and so on. On days when you're not feeling as motivated as you'd like, the calendar will showcase how much progress you've made and give you a push to keep going.

Exercise: Detox Calendar

Using the sample calendar from before as a model, you can make your own by following these simple steps.

1) List out all the days of the month using colored ink.

2) Describe what you wish to achieve under each day.

3) Leave room for listing side effects, improvements, or other notes as you wish.

4) Place it in the spot where you're most likely to see and update it daily.

Possible Side Effects

Now this is something worth mentioning when you begin your detox regimen, there is the possibility that you may experience some side effects.

Once again, you should always consult your physician before, during, and after a detox, but a few of the side effects listed below are to be expected.

- **Aches and pains:** Headaches, muscle, and joint pains are some of the symptoms you can expect due to rapid movement of toxins. The best thing to do when you experience this symptom is to have a good massage and a good sleep. It should get better over time.

- **Increased bathroom visits:** With a diet of mostly fluids and fiber, you may experience increased bowel movements and urination on your detox. This should return to normal after your detox.

- **More mucus:** The lymphatic tissue gets rid of mucus via the nose and throat, and experiencing this may make you concerned that you have a cold. Symptoms should clear up once you're finished with your detox.

- **Bloating:** With lots of fruit intake, you may experience bloating and gas. This usually occurs for the first few days of your detox but should subside as your body gets used to the new diet system. If it doesn't, cut down on your fruit intake until symptoms subside.

CHAPTER 6

Fresh Start to a Healthier Life

Detoxing is a very important part of living. Just like an engine will clog up and needs cleaning, the body also needs a washing after working for a while.

There are various organs involved in taking out waste from the body, including the skin, liver, and kidneys. While these organs work hard to take out waste, a small amount of toxins are always left behind, leaving the rest up to you to further assist your body to remove them.

Everyone should carry out a detox program a few times every year.

With everything that has been discussed, it should be now easy to pick the detox that's right for you. Whether you want to target an organ or a symptom, following the outlined steps will leave you with a refreshed feeling and renewed confidence in your health.

Detox Cleanse Express

Now You Know!

We have now gone from - *NOT knowing*...to *KNOWING*.

Doesn't it feel great? As cliché as the proverbial saying goes:
knowledge is, indeed, power. The more you know, the
more empowered you become. Not knowing is defeating,
as you succumb to feelings of helplessness and surrendering
of your own self.

Of course, acquiring knowledge is a never-ending quest.
There is a great saying by Nobel Prize French author
Andre Gide: "Believe those who are seeking the truth.
Doubt those who find it."

At the very least, we hope we have set you off in the right
path in regards to what you have set out to know, and that

you have enjoyed our little journey together for the time you have spent with us.

If you can tell us how we did, that would be very appreciated! We value your feedback and always look forward to hearing from you, or if there is any way we could improve the entire experience for you. If you have a success story, even better - please let us know!

http://www.KnowItExpress.com

Don't forget to stay in contact for we would love to connect with you.

https://www.facebook.com/KnowItExpress
https://twitter.com/KnowItExpress
https://plus.google.com/+KnowItExpress

What would you like to know? Let us know!

CONTACT US

Now onward for more power to you, and thank you!